Yoga for Beginners

*The Modern Guide of Yoga Poses for Beginners to Practice
Yoga and Meditation in Less than 24 Hours*

Yoga for Beginners

The Modern Guide of Yoga Poses for Beginners to Practice Yoga and Meditation in Less than 24 Hours

By: Robert Junior

© Copyright 2015 Robert Junior

Preface

First of all, let me tell you that you really need to be very happy for downloading my book. ***"The Modern Guide of Yoga Poses for Beginners to Practice Yoga and Meditation in Less than 24 Hours"***.

Inside this handy little book you will find proven steps and strategies on how to learn the basics about yoga and through the practice of it learn the art of meditation, lower your stress levels, lose weight, become fitter and improve the overall level of your living conditions.

Throughout this book I am going to analyze in great detail many tips and tricks you can use in order not only to get in control of the whole thing but stay in control for the years to come.

As long as you follow the steps and guidelines you will read in this book I can guarantee you that you are going to see the first actual results and feel the difference within weeks.

This book will provide a lot of details on what is yoga, why is it important to practice it, how to be a yoga practitioner, in what aspects of your life you are going to see major improvement and how to stay on track in order to achieve your goals as fast as possible.

Thanks again for downloading this book, I hope you enjoy it!

What Others Have To Say

☆☆☆☆☆ **A perfect mini-guide to yoga**, January 15, 2015

By **Terry Ward** - See all my reviews

Verified Purchase (What's this?)

This review is from: **Yoga: The Step By Step Guide of Yoga Poses for Beginners To Practice Meditation, Manage Stress and Lose Weight (Yoga, Yoga For Beginners, Meditation, Health, Stress Management) (Kindle Edition)**

My friend has been trying to talk me into taking a yoga class with her and though I've heard that it's very beneficial I felt a bit reluctant. I bought this book in order to get a little more information about yoga and what I could expect from a class. This book taught me exactly what I needed to know about yoga. Not too much....but just enough. I appreciated that it talked about what you could expect in your first yoga class. It also taught me more on the benefits of yoga and gave examples of stretches I could expect.

☆☆☆☆☆ **This book is a must read for anyone who wants to study or practice yoga**, January 15, 2015

By **Stuart Powell** - See all my reviews

Verified Purchase (What's this?)

This review is from: **Yoga: The Step By Step Guide of Yoga Poses for Beginners To Practice Meditation, Manage Stress and Lose Weight (Yoga, Yoga For Beginners, Meditation, Health, Stress Management) (Kindle Edition)**

Absolutely fantastic! I adore this book! I have tried for years to commit to yoga and taking care of myself and this book finally gave me the best motivation to do just that! It explains yoga in the clearest way! I got so much from this book and many of its messages have stayed with me since reading it. It's definitely something I'll re-read at different times, and it's already had an impact on how I see things. It is amazing.

☆☆☆☆☆ **Perfect Guide To Starting Yoga**, January 17, 2015

By **Wai Ka Liu** (San Francisco) - See all my reviews

Verified Purchase (What's this?)

This review is from: **Yoga: The Step By Step Guide of Yoga Poses for Beginners To Practice Meditation, Manage Stress and Lose Weight (Yoga, Yoga For Beginners, Meditation, Health, Stress Management) (Kindle Edition)**

Yoga is a great exercise not only for your body but for the mind. I've always wanted to get into yoga, but never knew where to start. I always thought it may be difficult to get started but after reading this book, it gave me a better sense of knowledge around yoga. This book had easy to follow sections and images making it very easy start. I recommend this book all that is interested in starting yoga.

☆☆☆☆☆ **Benefits of Yoga and Meditation**, January 19, 2015

By **Sophie** - See all my reviews

Verified Purchase (What's this?)

This review is from: **Yoga: The Step By Step Guide of Yoga Poses for Beginners To Practice Meditation, Manage Stress and Lose Weight (Yoga, Yoga For Beginners, Meditation, Health, Stress Management) (Kindle Edition)**

A well written guide on yoga with pictures of various yoga poses. In today's world the word stress is very common and even small age chidren are stressed with one or many reasons. Our eating and sleeping habits are completely out of order and so diseases are increasing a lot.

Yoga and meditation are proven techniques to lower down stress level, loose weight, become fitter and improve the overall level of our living condition. One can have benefit in all aspects of life from having a sharp memory to a fit muscular body. Just try it for a month and results can be seen

☆☆☆☆☆ **Great Beginner Guide**, January 15, 2015

By **Kristina Newman** - See all my reviews

Verified Purchase (What's this?)

This review is from: **Yoga: The Step By Step Guide of Yoga Poses for Beginners To Practice Meditation, Manage Stress and Lose Weight (Yoga, Yoga For Beginners, Meditation, Health, Stress Management) (Kindle Edition)**

As someone that is new to yoga I was looking for a step by step guide to learn the practice. I want to start taking classes at my gym but wanted to learn as much as I could at home before hand. This book was just what I was looking for. I liked this book a lot, it was a lot easier to understand compared to other yoga guides that I've just purchased. I highly recommend this book to anyone else that is just starting out learning Yoga.

☆☆☆☆☆ **Yoga for Me and You**, January 15, 2015

By **Mariana** - See all my reviews

Verified Purchase (What's this?)

This review is from: **Yoga: The Step By Step Guide of Yoga Poses for Beginners To Practice Meditation, Manage Stress and Lose Weight (Yoga, Yoga For Beginners, Meditation, Health, Stress Management) (Kindle Edition)**

Yoga is a system of exercises for mental and physical health. I've been wondering how yoga is done? Especially on mental exercise. Thank you for this informative book. Surely, it will help for those who are new in yoga. Though before I used to meditate and I thought I'm already doing yoga but still I know their is lacking doing it. Now, I can say 95% ~ 100% I can perform it well.

☆☆☆☆☆ **Its a very good book and also extremely analytical**, January 16, 2015

By **katerina Gior** - See all my reviews

Verified Purchase (What's this?)

This review is from: **Yoga: The Step By Step Guide of Yoga Poses for Beginners To Practice Meditation, Manage Stress and Lose Weight (Yoga, Yoga For Beginners, Meditation, Health, Stress Management) (Kindle Edition)**

Yoga is an incredible mean of calm and communication with our inner self and and spirit harmony,you can expel all negative influences,you can exercise and relax at the same time,tone your body.Its a very good book and also extremely analytical. Meditation is the part that i loved a lot,i've done some exercise for a few seconds by breathing the way the book says and some other exercises and i saw that its very effective.
My advice....begin reading and do some good for yourself!!!!

☆☆☆☆☆ **... wanted to do Yoga but just can't find a perfect time for it**, January 18, 2015

By **Kryzty Mae** - See all my reviews

Verified Purchase (What's this?)

This review is from: **Yoga: The Step By Step Guide of Yoga Poses for Beginners To Practice Meditation, Manage Stress and Lose Weight (Yoga, Yoga For Beginners, Meditation, Health, Stress Management) (Kindle Edition)**

I've always wanted to do Yoga but just can't find a perfect time for it. But this year, I'm going to see to it to join a yoga class. I've heard a lot of good things about doing yoga and it's positive effects. The one reason why I purchased this book is so I could have an idea on yoga poses since this is really my first time to do this. This book contains everything I need to know about yoga and yoga posses. This is a perfect book for beginners like me.

Table Of Contents

Table of Contents

Getting Started

The word 'Yoga' derives from the word 'yuj' in Sanskrit, meaning 'to unite.' This is appropriate given the multitude of purposes that yoga serves. Aside from the core reality that like-minded people from around the world come together quite often to share in its experience, yoga itself represents the unity of many different principles that can serve our everyday needs.

If you're reading this book you've already taken a step in the right direction. Yoga not only helps the practitioner get into better physical shape, it's a holistically beneficial activity. This book is going to help you approach yoga as a beginner and give you some tips to succeed in your quest for a better mind, spirit and body, which is what the practice of yoga is all about. Yoga's benefits are innumerable.

It's important to first dispel some of the myths about yoga. Despite being an activity that is sometimes associated with the feminine, there are many males that participate in the practice and there are a high number of male teachers. Some types of yoga, such as Hatha Flow, the most popular, are quite strenuous; enough so that it should instantly debunk any myths about yoga is too girly an activity for blustery males. Some also tend to believe that you need to be flexible to do yoga. This is patently untrue. Many yogis are not flexible at all, though the practice encourages them to expand their flexibility over time. Part of the rationale of yoga is accepting that bodies are unique and different. Respecting the limitations of your body is key and is also important in avoiding injury.

First let's discuss the body. Yoga has rejuvenating effects that surprise even veterans. A standard class lasts one and a half hours, and classes are often very strenuous. Yet at the end of them, yogis do not feel emptied of energy but just the opposite. Rather, they quite often feel energetic and ready for their day. Yoga classes are typically held throughout the day, running from as early as 5am to 7pm at night. Exercises are also extremely balanced, meaning that they practically focus on the body as a whole, rather than just one small part. In this book, students of yoga are referred to as 'yogis.' Experienced employees leading the class are simply called 'teachers' or 'yoga teachers.'

Avoiding Injury

Yoga is a very safe activity, as the entire practice typically takes place on a solitary mat. I can't really stress enough the importance of a Yoga mat as new students sometimes overlook this. A very economic, yet high quality Yoga mat I have already found is this one. However an in any physical endeavor, especially involving strenuous exercise, there is a risk of overdoing things and injuring yourself. Here are a few ways not to do that. First, yoga should generally be avoided by women in the late stages of pregnancy. Generally at this point many of the poses are difficult to begin with. Also if there are prior injuries it's possible to exacerbate them. Yoga places a lot of pressure on the feet and the wrists. It isolates different parts of the body generally, and focuses on them one by one. Yogis with prior injuries in these areas could make things worse. Generally in the beginning of the class instructors will ask their students if they have prior injuries. It's important to be honest with them. If you ever need to take a break, particularly if in the course of the practice you are putting pressure on an area that makes you physically uncomfortable, there is nothing wrong with taking a break and going into the child's pose. You can wait there until the focus shifts to another body part. Some of the more challenging poses can be worrisome if the yogi does not have control. Beginners should be careful for instance when they try head stands and shoulder stands in the first few months of their practice. Generally a spotter is required to prevent balance from being lost, which could end up causing a cascade of teetering yogis, knocking each other over like dominos across the room.

Yoga etiquette

It's important to maintain yoga etiquette if you're going to a public class. It's not as if you'll be inundated by tons of different rules, but there are a few basic expectations that it's important to be aware of. The first of these is that you generally want to be early to class, so you have time to set up your mat (or a borrowed one) and get into a relaxed state. Class members sometimes chat when they first arrive, but as it becomes time to begin they are generally expected to fall silent and become attentive to the instructor. Bathroom breaks are fine, but are not all that common. The sessions are rather long (1.5 hours) so it's permissible to leave, but if you do just make sure not to disrupt the class. Some yoga centers may ask that males not take their shirts off during practice or that yogis avoid showing up already emanating unpleasant odors. This may seem strange given that yoga is a highly physical activity, but it's also meant to appeal to the other senses, including smell. There is generally incense burning in the room, so as to make for a pleasant aroma.

The Origin Of Yoga

While yoga is a modern activity, it is in fact an ancient practice that has been developing for many centuries in tandem with Hinduism. It celebrates some of the main Hindu beliefs, including those of peace, serenity and harmony with both mankind and nature, the destruction of the ego and a mental flow state that encourages creativity, positivity and originality. Adherence to discipline is also a key belief, as yogis are encouraged to endure the physical and mental hardship of practice for the duration of the class as best they can.

Yoga originates from the Indus civilization, which encompassed 300,000 square miles in part of what is now modern India. Sources differ on the precise date that the practice of yoga began, as this goes back so long that it's difficult to say. There is proof however that yoga has been in practice for at least 5,000 years, based upon depictions of figures in yogic poses in the cities of Daro, Harappa and Mohenjo found by archaeologists. Yet there are indications that yoga may have been in existence for possibly even up to 17,000 years. This has led to a deep, wise and streamlined practice that has stood the test of time.

Just because the practice has been around for so long doesn't necessarily mean that it has always existed in the form that it's in today. It has gone through many different permutations throughout its long journey before it became popular in western civilization. In fact, Hatha, which is perhaps the most pervasive form of yoga today, was created in the 4th and 5th centuries, and took centuries to become culturally relevant around the world. Many practitioners and gurus (or teachers) who have decided to make yoga a top priority in their lives have gone to India to practice, where yoga is taught in a manner that is considered the closest to its purest form possible.

Teacher training is popular in India as well and often linked closely to lengthy sessions of vows of silence and meditation. Travelers have found India to be a spectacular destination; though it is one with which many yogis have a love/hate relationship. It is both one of the most beautiful travel destinations in the world and one of the most challenging, especially during attempts to explore the 'real India', outside the comfort of tourist zones and luxury. Learning more about the origin of yoga will enrich your experience, and put you in touch with the fundamental principles, which can be life changing additions to its physical benefits.

The Standard Format

This chapter discusses the many different forms of yoga to help guide the reader in deciding where to start, and eventually how to manage his or her time when it comes to your personal practice. It should be noted that although most yoga centers also sometimes offer alternative classes like Salsa and Pilates. This is simply because yogis are often interested in these activities as well, and some yoga teachers have skills in both.

While differing in terms of difficulty and style most yoga classes have a similar format. Generally students begin seated on their mats facing the front of the room with their legs crossed. In yoga etiquette all participants usually fall silent and place their attention on the instructor. Talking during the practice is usually limited, although from time to time the instructor will ask whether the students have questions. If there's an emergency of course it's fine to bring an interruption. Aside from this talking during the session on the part of the participants should be generally kept to a minimum. Hands rest on the knees with palms facing upward. Some yogis extend their fingers or put them in a ring configuration, while others just rest them there. Instructors will sometimes come around the room and help the participants by adjusting their posture. Some instructors make a point of asking yogis who are uncomfortable being touched to signify this somehow, usually by turning one corner of their mat under. If you prefer this boundary, this is an option.

The teacher will also ask the participants to sit up as straight as possible and tilt their heads slightly back. At first this can be difficult, particularly for participants who are accustomed to slouching. Over time however one becomes accustomed to this pose, and it makes a giant improvement to posture, which helps maintain the health of the back over the long term. Different teachers have different styles. Some prefer to give speeches at the beginning of the session. These often adhere to different themes, like positivity, discipline or perseverance and are designed to share some of the ancient spoken wisdom that comes from the practice of yoga. Other teachers prefer not to talk much in the beginning and get right into the practice. Before the physical activity begins there is a session of ohms, when participants are asked to mimic the teacher's sounds vocally. This tends to put the class in sync. Generally this is short as well. If you don't feel comfortable participating verbally you aren't required to do so, but in order to get the full experience of the session participants are usually encouraged to trust the leadership of the instructor.

Classes typically start with easier stretches that are integrated into the program. Stretching in the beginning is not like stretching before a sports practice. It's part of the fabric of yoga itself. This may seem strange but if participants simply follow the instruction of the teacher it is made easy. Instructors often mimic the poses that they ask their students to do to give examples. If a student is having difficulty getting into a pose, an instructor will generally step over and help guide him or her. This is quite common too with handstands and headstands, which are some of the more difficult and precarious positions in yoga. When a yogi is guided by a spotter they become much easier. Then over time students can learn to do these poses on their own.

Although not always performing strenuous activity throughout the entirety of the practice, participants are always kept more or less 'busy' or occupied. There are no real breaks but there are periodic resting times where the child's pose is used, most often just after the most strenuous portions of the practice. Usually in the beginning the pace is slow, and it often begins to speed up significantly about twenty minutes into the practice. Some poses focus on the legs (or one leg at a time) while others focus on the upper body. Often there are variations of a pose based upon relative difficulty, and these are described by the instructor to allow the students to choose the pose that suits them best.

Periodic breaks are given throughout. Near the end of the practice instructors resort to 'cool down' poses which are intended to bring the body back into a state of rest and relaxation. Practice ends with the savasana, in which the students lie on their backs, usually for about five to ten minutes to the sound of soothing music or silence. This is a kind of meditation period in which chants or relaxing words are spoken by the instructor. After the savasana, students sit up again as in the beginning of the practice session with their legs crossed, arms resting on their knees, and palms open upward. Chants are repeated again.

Showing Up

It may be a little intimidating showing up to your first yoga class, so this chapter fleshes out what the experience is like to show fresh yogis that yoga studios are casual environments. Remember also that you're there to maintain a state of low stress. You want to get a workout in and possibly to engage in meditation. Anxiety is the last thing you should want to experience. If you're feeling out of shape, don't compare your body to others'. Yoga is supposed to be all about self-improvement, and while some yogis are particularly proud of their achievements, communities are generally very welcoming. That said there seldom needs to be any conversing involved before class begins. Plenty of yogis prefer to set up their mats silently without talking to anyone, as a way to prepare themselves mentally for practice.

The teacher may ask the yogis to raise their hands if it is their first class. This happens more often in difficult classes, where there can be concern that a beginner has mistakenly wandered into a class too advanced for him or her. Despite its reputation as a primarily feminine activity, yoga can be an incredibly strenuous activity, pushing the limits of one's physical cardio, balance and longevity.

Before you go, check the schedule to see if the classes are numbered in terms of difficulty. It's recommended that beginners start out with at least one 'intro' class. That way they can broadly and slowly introduce themselves to the different core poses without feeling the pressure of quick transitions, which are often quite difficult even for very experienced yogis.

Beginners should always remember that if they get too tired to keep up with the rest of the class during session, it's perfectly fine to return to the 'child's position', which is designed for rest. Teachers should introduce this early-on to beginners. The chin is tucked in while the knees are bent and tucked into the chest. Toes are pointed while the body leans forward on the legs. This pose is not always comfortable at first, but becomes comfortable with time.

Some beginners are worried about needing equipment for yoga, but this is not the case. That's one of the beauties of this practice. All you need to do is show up wearing workout gear. For ladies a pushup bra and yoga pants are fine, but gym shorts work just as well. Some yogis make a point of their yoga fashion getup. If that's part of a ritual that adds meaning to the practice for you, then it's certainly worth it. But having special yoga pants isn't going to give you a better workout. What's more important is your attentiveness and adherence to the teacher's direction, your breathing and self-awareness, your developing agility and balance, and your self-improvement over time. For those that really care about the core significance of yoga, fashion is a superficial element. It is sometimes helpful to remember that Lululemon didn't exist thousands of years ago in India where yoga was developed, when fashion in yoga was less of a priority. Don't scrutinize your clothes as much as you do your technique and commitment. This doesn't mean that yogis should feel bad if they can't go every day, but focus in the moment is a key priority.

As for mats, they are made available for use already, so you can just borrow them at the studio. You don't need any other equipment. Just bring your body and a positive attitude. Aside from that, you're ready to go! Happy practice!

Popular Types of Yoga

The following forms of yoga are some of the most popular. Take a look below to see what you think might fit you best in getting started out. Naturally over the long term it is healthy to expand your horizons and try new forms of yoga as much as possible. You never know. It could become your favorite new thing! Descriptions include difficulty levels along with the general focus of the class.

Hatha (Flow)

Hatha focuses on body movements designed to break a sweat through compound exercises that divide the body into quarters. Generally it has a heavy focus on building leg strength and leg balance at the same time, transitioning then into an upper-body focus, which includes push-up like motions in short repetition. Ordinary hatha classes focus on holding one or more positions for longer periods of time whereas hatha flow classes feature more rapid movement for the purpose of getting a more active workout.

Vinyasa (Flow)

Vinyasa classes are a form of Hatha yoga designed to focus on the more physical aspect of yogic exercise within the standard format of a yoga class, including chants in the beginning and a savasana at the end. The core format is for participants to periodically come to rest in the downward dog position, sometimes transitioning back to plank, then leaping with the feet forward such that they're positioned next to the hands. The next step is to reach the hands high up in the air, then down again to the feet, leap backwards, then drop the body down in a push-up fashion to the ground yet without making full contact with the chest. Pushing the body up again as the legs are straight and the feet are pointing backwards, the body transitions into downward dog and then plank position. This process begins slow and gradually increases in speed. Other stretches and exercises are integrated, but generally this routine is what gives the practice its continuity.

Meditation

While many classes are quite physically active, others focus almost entirely on meditation and on linking meditation to breathing exercises. Those who do not meditate on a regular basis will want to start with a lower level class, as the higher level classes often require that participants meditate for longer periods of time. Generally, the meditation sessions in beginner level classes last for around fifteen minutes with some occasional physical exercises to stretch out the body and create some contrast during the class. Meditation focuses on relaxing the body completely and exiting all thoughts from the mind, striving to attain a new height of focus and consciousness. Teachers often guide participants through different mantras that help one to attain this state of mind.

Readers should remember that there are many different kinds of meditation as well. Some focus particularly on the release of physical and emotional pain, involving a chance for venting. Students are generally encouraged not just to meditate during class, but at home as well. 10 minutes of meditation every day can make a huge difference, and change one's perspective on life.

Breathing Classes

Breathing classes are often held in yoga centers. These include a variety of different techniques, which try to heighten consciousness through rapid breathing, circular breathing, and the syncopation of breathing with different physical exercises. Breathing exercises border on a kind of hyperventilation, which can be exhilarating, and rehabilitating with respect to the mind and consciousness. The beauty of these exercises is that once learned they can be done nearly anywhere.

Pilates

Although not technically yoga, and developed much more recently, pilates exercises share many of the same movements and concepts as yoga, with a focus on developing the muscles in the core, enhancing balance, breathing, and centering exercises. The concept of centering derives from understanding the core as being the center of intent and identity aside from just the development of the abdominal muscles. Pilates is more an exercise-centric activity than yoga, which embodies a more spiritual aspect.

Core Positions and Progression

You'll learn these if you take a beginner's class, but just to familiarize the reader with them, here are some of the core positions in yoga. These are generally the first things that a beginner learns when he or she comes to class. It's important to do these with correct technique. Otherwise, not only can this be harmful to parts of your body, but your muscle memory could develop the wrong habits, which is not the best path for advancement!

Downward Dog

In this position the yogi is facing downward (true to its name), supported by both hands and feet in what should look essentially like an upside down 'V'. The back should be straight while the arms are outstretched forward and parallel to each other. Harm can come to the wrists by being in this position while the wrists are rotated inward or outward. Yogis should try to move their feet closer to their hands. Some try to flatten their feet, though this is not possible for some. At first this is a difficult pose to hold for long periods of time. However later on it becomes a comfortable spot for resting.

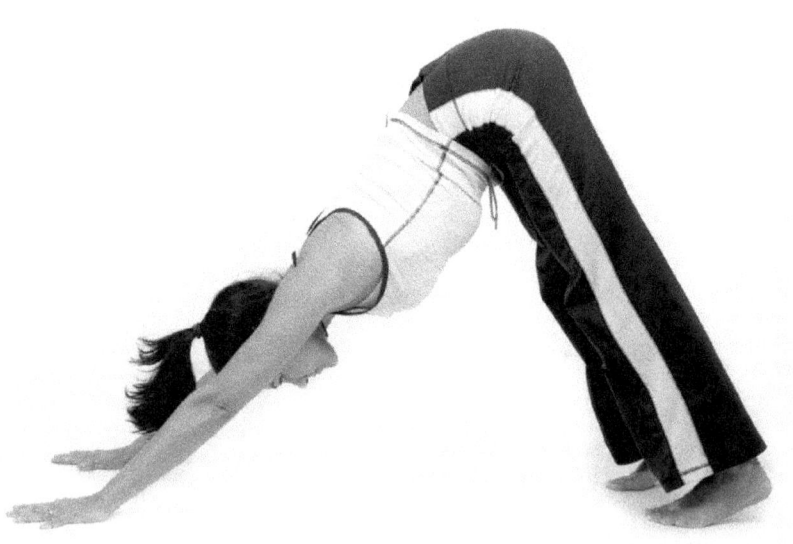

Warrior Pose (1, 2 & 3)

The warrior pose begins with one leg extended out in front of the body, foot flat on the floor and knee at a right angle, while the other leg is extended backwards and remains straight. The back leg is supported by standing on the toes. Meanwhile the arms are outstretched in the direction consistent with legs i.e. right leg forward, right arm forward, left leg backward, left arm backward. This describes the warrior pose 1. Usually afterward this transitions into warrior pose 2, in which the only thing that changes is that the hands move to being outstretched at the sides. In warrior pose 3 the back foot is lifted up into the air such that the balance is kept on only the front foot while both arms remain outstretched to the sides. This works out the solo leg in addition to being a challenging balance exercise. Moving through these phases with finesse and control is also part of the challenge, as is letting the airborne foot down gradually and softly.

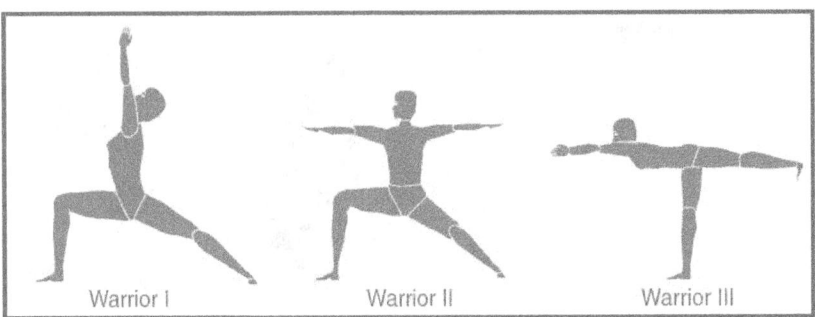

Warrior I   Warrior II   Warrior III

Cat-Cow Stretch

This begins on the hands and knees, head facing upward and back facing straight. It transitions to the head facing down and the back arching. This is considered a way of opening up the heart and loosening up the mid-section. This is also a core position from which the legs can be extended one by one, testing endurance. A more advanced variation involves lifting the hand on the opposite side of your body and outstretching it forward or straight to the side. This manifests a challenge for balance as well.

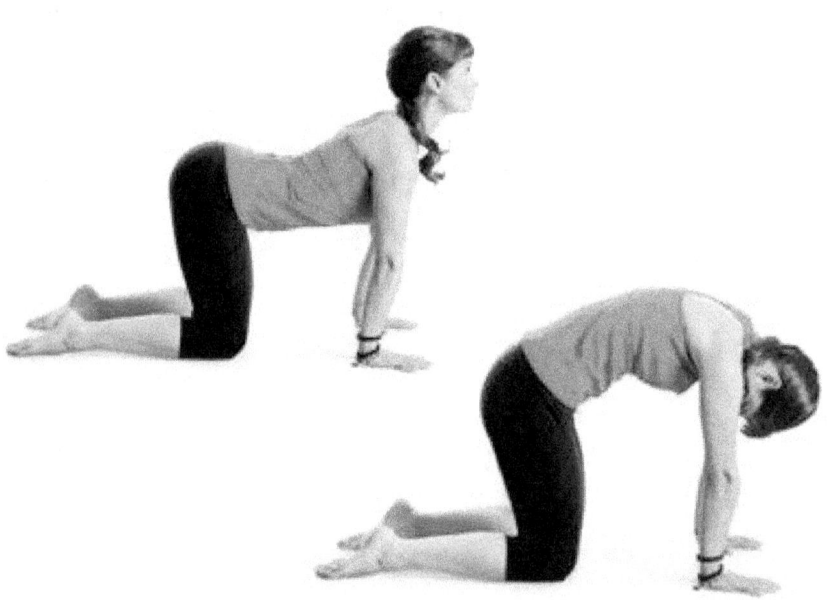

Child's Pose

Child's pose is excellent for stretching out your lower back and realigning your discs, as well as stretching and strengthening your hips. This pose is used to relieve stress, abdominal upset, fatigue, and lower back discomfort. If you're someone who sits in a chair all day at work, then you would benefit from Child's Pose. To perform the pose, you would sit on your heels with your hands on your thighs and lower your chest to the rest on your thighs. Bring your forehead down to the floor and relax your arms beside your legs with your palms facing the ceiling. Hold this pose for five to ten deep breaths and then slowly sit up. If you still feel tight in your back or you're still stressed, try to meditate while in this pose.

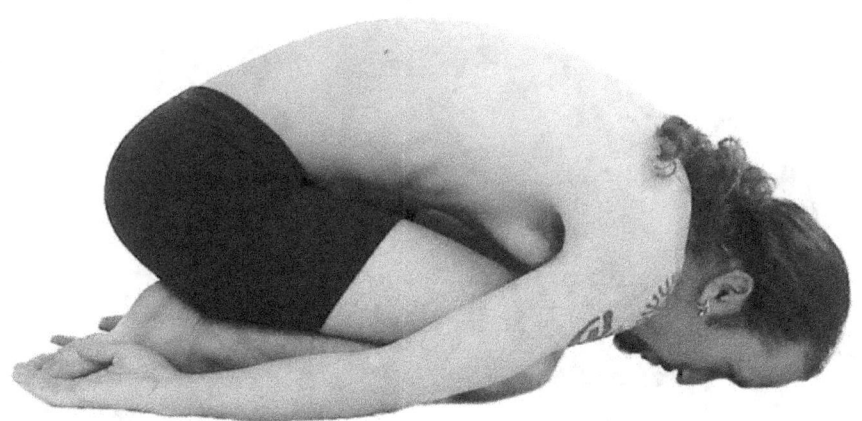

Child's Pose, Wide-Kneed Variation

Sometimes you need to perform a pose that's a little more widening to help you stretch your lower and upper back muscles, as well as your hips, thighs, and groin area. If you're experiencing indigestion or a scattered mind, the wide-kneed variation of child's pose is an excellent one to start with. Simply get into position for downward-facing dog. Now lift your heels and separate your knees while you lower down to the floor. Lower your body to the mat and keep your hands stretched in front of you instead of beside you. Your knees should be a little bit apart and your arms stretched out straight.

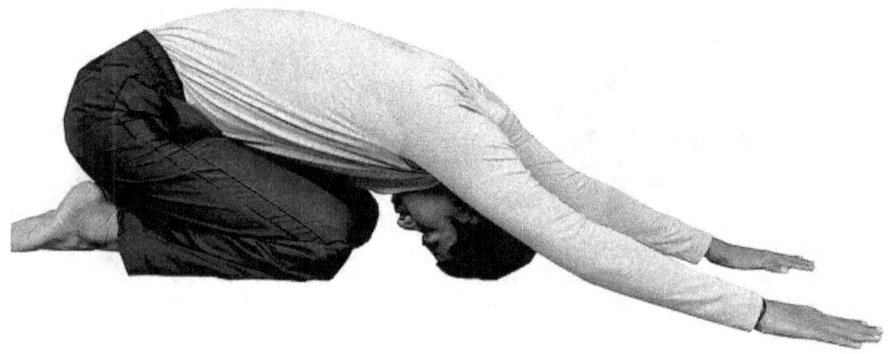

Knees to Chest

The knees to chest position is excellent for beginners and helps relieve digestive upset as well as relieve stress. If you have a tight back, then you should do this pose. To perform the pose, lie down on your back and put your feet flat on the floor with your knees bent. Your arms should be stretched out beside your body with your palms facing up. Bring your knees to your chest and place your right hand on your right shin as well as your left hand on your left shin. Pull you knees toward you. Wrap your arms around your legs until the inside of your elbows are touching your legs, and then grasp hold of your right elbow with your left hand and your left elbow with your right hand. Rock back and forth ten times gently and then release your elbows. Keep your right hand on your right knee and your left hand on your left knee, and make ten circles with your legs and hips. Keep the legs together.

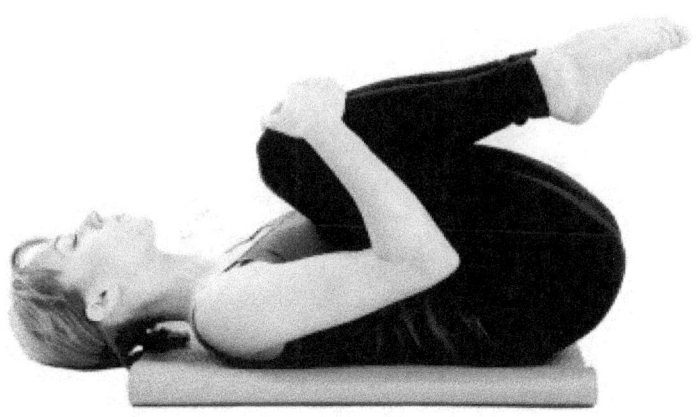

Legs Up The Wall

If you have tight hamstrings, chest, abs, and neck muscles, then the legs up the wall position will be good for you. People who suffer from tired legs and feet, anxiety, insomnia, stress, and a scattered mind should perform this position. To do the position, start by sitting with your knees bent and the left side of your body up against the wall. Place your palms on the floor beside your hips and turn your hips so that they're facing the wall while you swing your legs up. Your head should be back and your legs should be touching the wall. Place your buttocks against the wall so that you're straight. Hold for five to ten deep breaths.

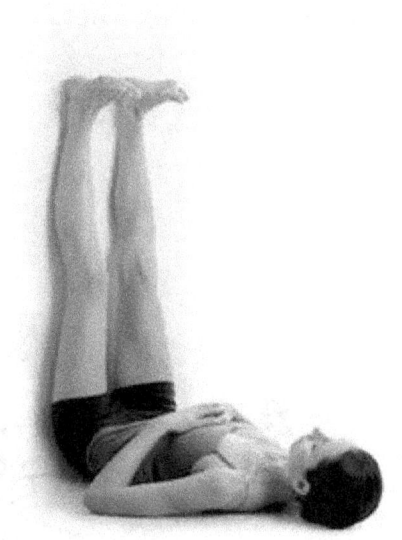

Mountain Pose

The mountain pose has to be one of the easiest physical poses out there in yoga, but you have to have a focused mind while you do it. It's for strengthening your back, legs, abs, and spine. People who have poor posture and a scattered mind should try this pose. Simply stand with your feet together and your big toes touching. You should be looking forward and not down. Now, tighten your thigh muscles, active your kneecaps, broaden your collarbone and stretch your arms down alongside your body. Hold for five to ten deep breaths.

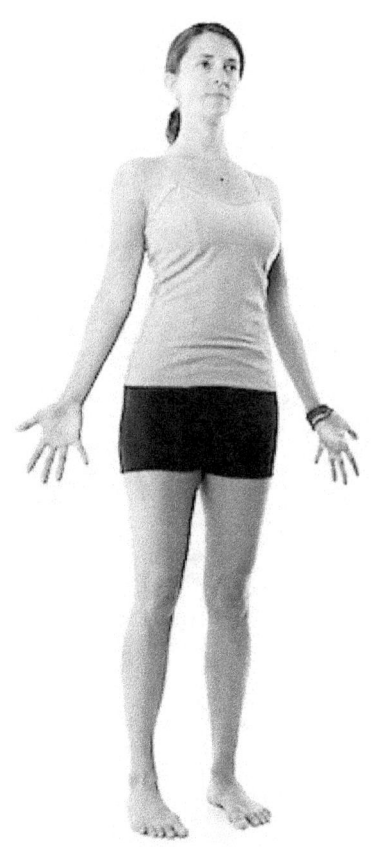

Reclining Twist

The reclining twist is also great for stretching your back, thighs, neck, glutes, and spine. Lie down on your back and extend your arms out straight from your shoulders. Shift your hips to the right and cross your right thigh over your left thigh. Now lift your legs up into the air and pull your knees a little closer to your torso. Allow your legs to drop to the left as you look the right. Hold for five to ten breaths and then switch sides.

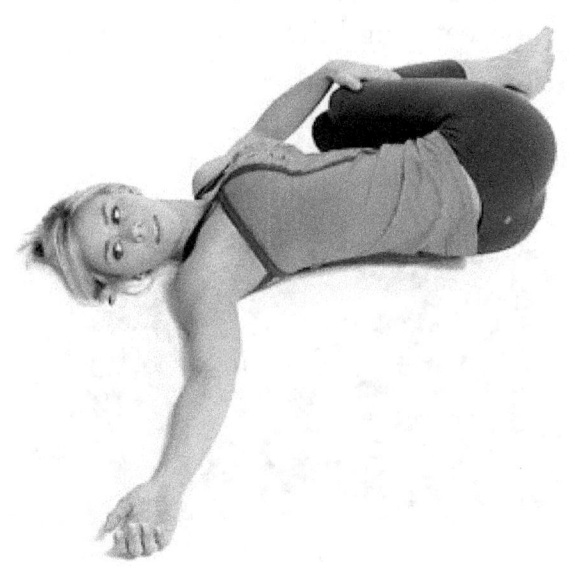

Seated Forward Bend

While it looks pretty easy, the seated forward bend is a little more difficult to perform if you're not very flexible. This is for stretching out your back, legs, and lengthening your spine. If you suffer from digestive upset and headaches, try this move. Sit in staff position with your legs out in front of you, your ankles touching, and your back and spine straight. Now inhale and place your arms above your head at shoulder width apart. Exhale and reach your arms forward until you can grasp hold of our toes, shins, or knees. Go only as far as you are comfortable. Lower your head between your shoulders or touch your forehead to your knees if you can. Hold this position for five breaths and then slowly sit up.

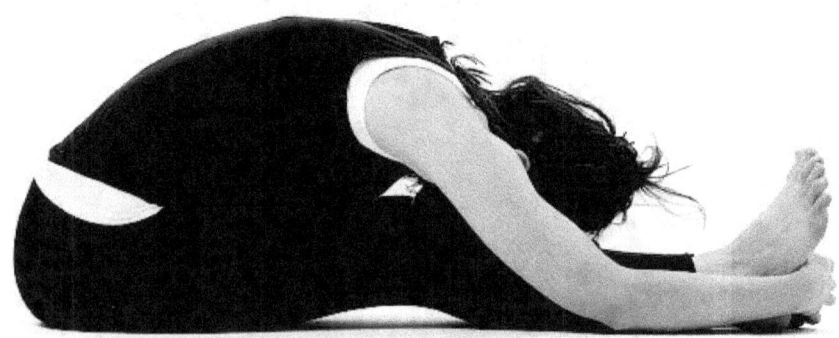

Seated Twist

The seated twist will stretch your hips and help with constipation or diarrhea. To perform this pose, sit in the agnistambhasana pose with your right foot on your left knee and your left foot on your right knee. Move your right leg with your hands and put the sole of your right foot on the floor next to your left knee. Your right toes should be facing forward. Now move your left foot back and bring the left heel next to your right hip. Extend your left arm up as you inhale, bend it and put your elbow and upper arm on the right side of your right knee. Put your right hand behind you. Place your left elbow into your right knee and twist your torso until your facing to the side. Put your left hand on the outside of your right hip to hold your position.

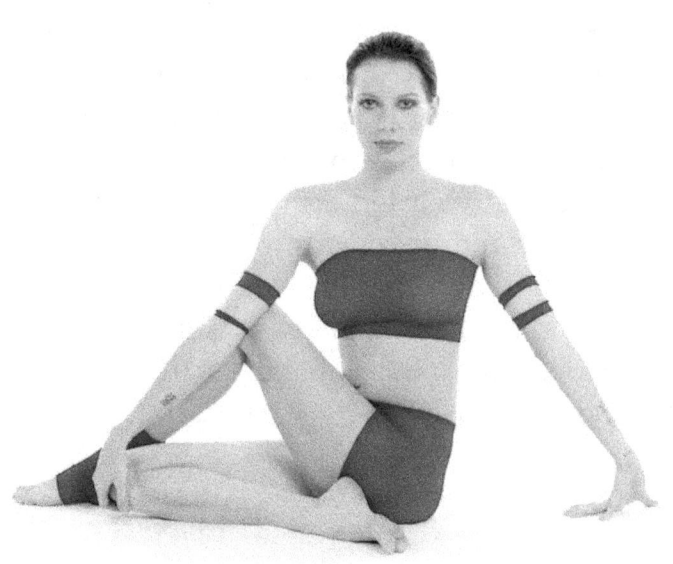

Sphinx Pose

The sphinx pose is great for stretching out your chest and your back. If you experience back pain, you should try this pose. Lie down with your front on the floor and your arms alongside your body with your palms facing up. Your forehead and toes should be on the floor. Lift your shoulders and chest and put your elbows under your shoulders in front of you on the floor. Let your forearms rest on the floor parallel to one another. Now press your palms into the floor and come into a slight backbend.

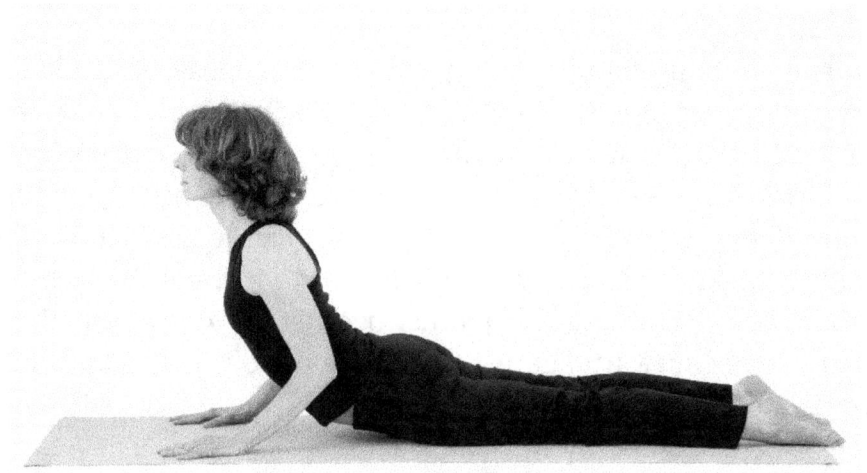

Squat Pose

Warning: You should not perform this pose if you are pregnant. Otherwise, the squat pose is excellent for strengthening your back, hips, thighs, and buttocks. To perform this pose, stand with your feet parallel and hip width apart. Turn your toes out at a forty-five degree angle and then bend your knees and lower your butt into a squat. Your torso should be upright and our palms together at your chest. Press your elbows outward against the inside of your knees and hold for five to ten breaths.

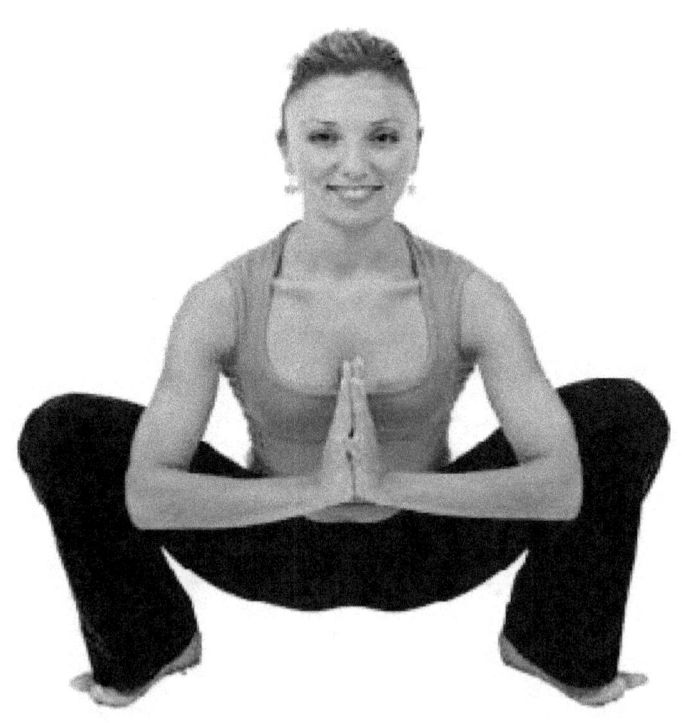

Staff Pose

Excellent for strengthening your thighs, core, and back, the staff pose is very easy to perform. Simply sit with your legs out in front of you and your ankles touching. Your toes should be pointing up. Place your hands next to your hips and slide your shoulder blades downward. Broaden your chest and reach forward through the inner edges of your feet and look straight ahead. Hold for five to ten deep breaths.

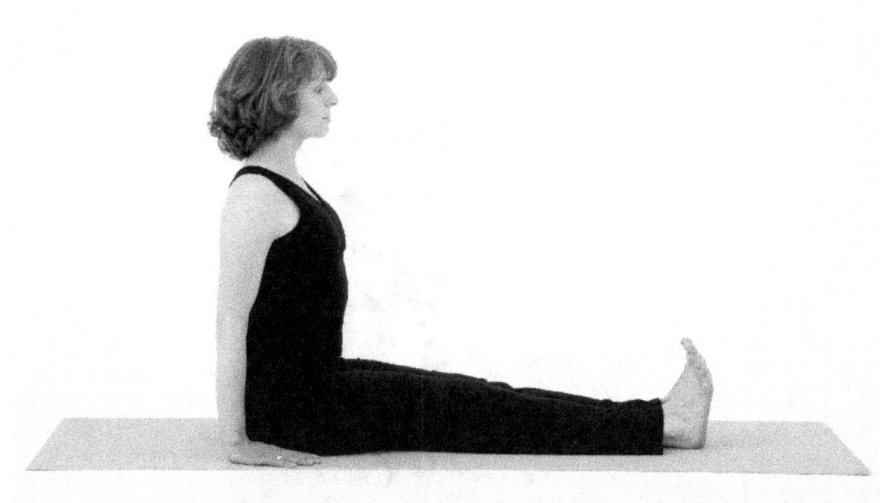

Standing Forward Bend

This might be considered one of the harder beginner moves because while it looks easy, it requires balance and flexibility. Start by standing in the mountain pose and bring your hands to a prayer position in front of you, palms together. Inhale and gaze up at the ceiling, lifting your chest as you do so. Then exhale and fold forward starting at the hips and keeping your spine straight. Do not allow your hips to get behind your ankles! Now bring your palms to the floor if you can, or fingertips, or grasp your shins if you must. Inhale and exhale five times, and then come back to the mountain pose.

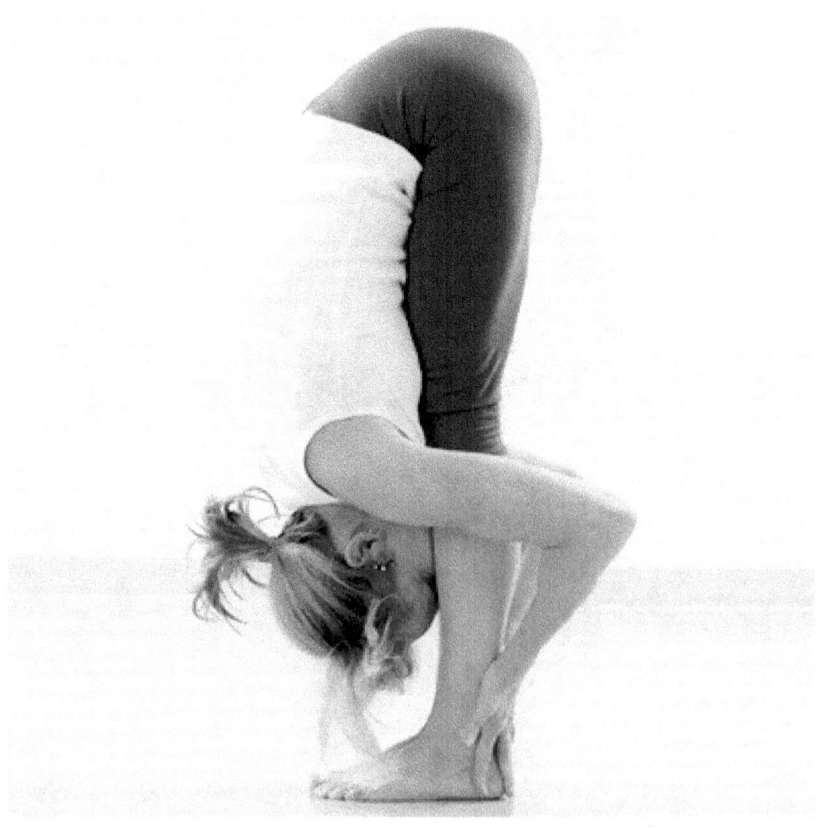

Savasana

The Savasana is the final pose in yoga, done at the end of every yoga practice. It is part resting, part meditation and part focusing on your purpose for the practice and on the effect you intend for it to have on your life. Though this is the least difficult pose of all physically, it has been said that there is no pose more difficult than the Savasana, because penetrating the core of its meaning involves a state of consciousness that requires unique experience and focus.

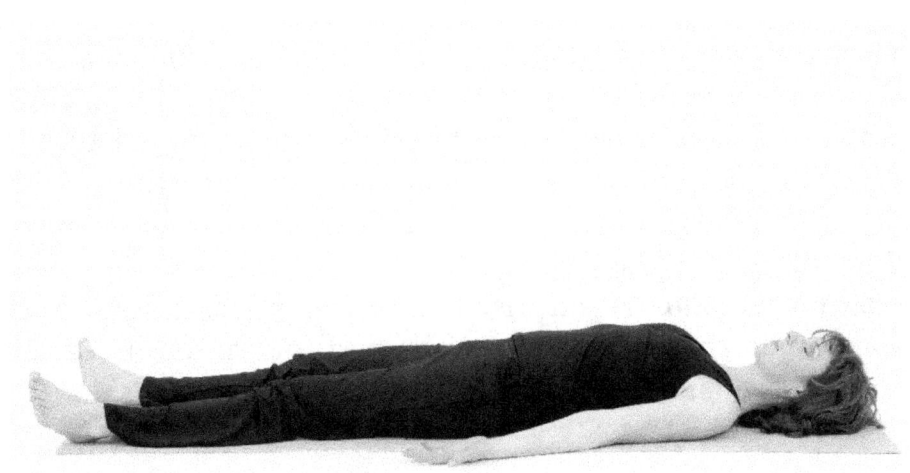

Progression

Now that you have a lot of the basics about yoga you'll be at an advantage when showing up to your first class. Let's talk a little bit about the process of progressing in yoga. Everyone tends to do so at their own pace, which depends not just on yoga but on consistently making healthy lifestyle choices, as in those that are conducive to your growth physically, mentally and spiritually. The great thing about yoga is that it puts you around people that tend to value healthy lifestyles. Their food choices and habits are likely to influence your own, and thus will result in even greater benefits over the long run.

There's an old saying that if you want to learn something fast, learn it slow, and if you want to learn it slow, learn it fast. Yoga is not a thing to be rushed, although when you do practice, it deserves your full attention and commitment. Those who periodically take breaks from yoga may also find that their time off has allowed them to process some of the body movements, and are surprised at how easy it is to return. If you simply commit to doing your best and go on a regular basis you will improve, and you're certain to see the results.

Conclusion

Thank you again for downloading this book! This section provides the conclusion. Just to keep the ideas fresh in your mind let's review what was discussed in the above chapters.

The first chapter introduced the concept of yoga, dispelled myths about the requirements to practice it, talked about how to stay safe and avoid injury, and briefly, yoga etiquette.

The second chapter covers what is needed for yoga class, mentions class difficulty and the child's pose, an important refuge for tired yogis, and dispels myths about importance of fashionable dress.

The third chapter discusses the nearly universal format of a yoga class to help beginners know what to expect when they come for the first time.

The fourth chapter briefly goes into the origin of yoga and its historical roots in India, which are important to remember in contemporary times.

The fifth chapter goes into more detail in describing the features of the core yoga classes. Some are more focused on meditation, while others on physical fitness.

The sixth chapter focused on describing the core positions in yoga and gives some final tips as to how progression is made.

I hope this book was able to help you to learn all you needed to know to get started with your yoga practice.

The next step is to not wait any longer in getting started with your yoga practice. It's a wonderfully beneficial activity, so sign up for a class today!

If you liked this eBook on Advanced Yoga Poses, please leave a positive review here. It will only take 1 minute but it is extremely important to me.

Thank you for reading!

With love and respect,

Robert Junior

Some Other Books From Us

Below you can find some of the other books published from us.

★**Preview Start**★

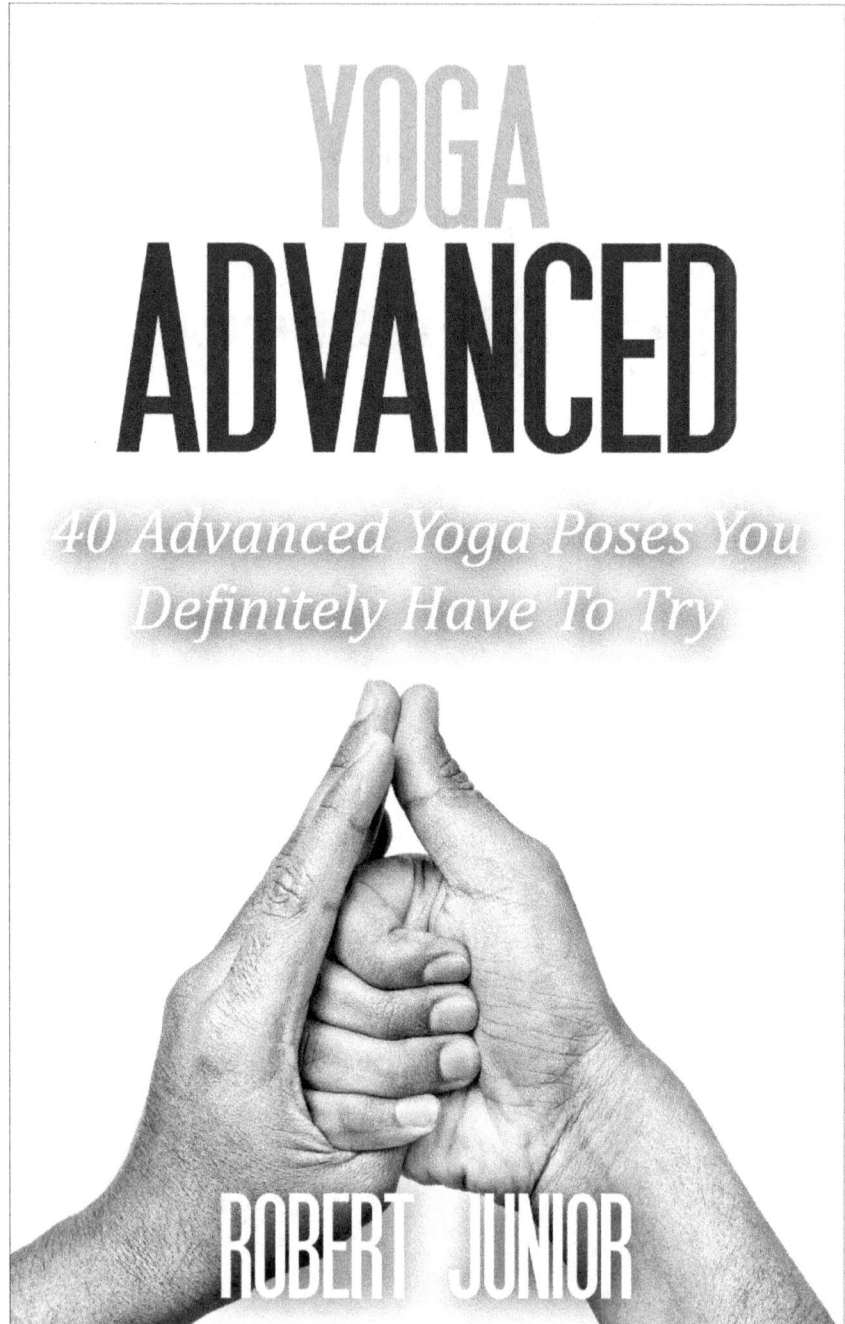

Preface

First of all, let me tell you how happy I am for downloading my book. *"**Advanced Yoga: 40 Advanced Yoga Poses - The Most Advanced and Simplified Yoga Guide on Earth**"*.

This book is the sequel of my first book of the series "Yoga for Beginners: The Modern Guide Of Yoga Poses for Beginners To Practice Meditation And Yoga In Less Than 24 Hours". If you enjoyed my first book...well this one is going to blow your mind away.

In this new sequel I have included over 40 advanced yoga poses that is the logical sequence of the first yoga poses for beginners. Hopefully by now you have mastered these easy poses and you are ready for your next step in the wonderful world of yoga.

Take control today, and come with me for a life-changing journey through the beautiful world of transcendence and mental awareness.

Thanks again for downloading this book, I hope you enjoy it!

Table of Contents

Firefly (★★★★★)

Fish (★★☆☆☆)

Forearm Balance (★★★★☆)

Frog (★★★☆☆)

Half Moon (★☆☆☆☆)

Handstand (★★★★☆)

Happy Baby (★★☆☆☆)

Headstand (★★★★★)

Locust (★★★★☆)

Locust Variation (★★★★☆)

Monkey (★★★★★)

One-Legged King Pidgeon (★★★★★)

Peacock (★★★★☆)

Pendant Pose (★★★★☆)

Plank (★★☆☆☆)

Plow (★★★★☆)

Rabbit (★★★★☆)

Reclining Hero (★☆☆☆☆)

Reverse Plank (★★★☆☆)

Reverse Warrior (★★★☆☆)

Shoulder Stand (★★★★☆)

Reference Poses

Warrior Pose II (★☆☆☆☆)

Pigeon Pose (★★★☆☆)

Conclusion

Introduction

If you're reading this book, you're most likely not a beginner at yoga. Therefore, I will briefly outline what you most likely already know. Yoga is more than a form of exercise. It is a lifestyle that people choose due to the mental, emotional, and physical benefits.

Some of the physical benefits include:

- Increased muscle strength, tone, flexibility, and balance.
- Increased vitality, energy, metabolism and improved respiration.
- Weight loss.
- Improved cardio health.
- And protection from injury.

Mental benefits include:

- The ability to manage stress.
- Development of coping skills.
- Develop a better outlook on life.

Emotional benefits include:

- Increased self-esteem.
- Ability to remain calm.

Before you begin with advanced yoga poses, let's take a look at some of the safety precautions you should take.

- Find an excellent, reputable instructor who is certified if you choose to practice within a classroom environment. They're knowledgeable about whether or not your body will be able to perform the poses they're displaying, and they should know what you can and cannot do if you have any type of injury or ailment.

- Do not treat yoga as a competition. This is a good way to get hurt while you're in a classroom or yoga environment because there are others out there who will be more advanced and flexible than you. If you push yourself too hard too fast, you risk injury.
- Be sure to stay within your limits. If you start to feel pain or severe discomfort, stop the pose immediately and go back to something easier.
- Warm-up before you begin. It's important to have your muscles loose and relaxed before you start twisting into poses. Cold muscles are more easily injured and less likely to be fluid enough to do intermediate poses. If you're comfortable with beginner poses, try doing a few of those before you slide into the intermediate poses.

Finally, what you'll need in order to practice the advanced poses within this book.

A quiet place. You'll want somewhere that you're not distracted because yoga is more than just physical, it's about the calmness of your mind.

A yoga mat or soft place outside. There's a possibility you may lose your balance with these poses, so having somewhere that you can get an easy grip and fall softly is a good idea.

A relaxed mental and physical state. Pretty self-explanatory, but you should be warm and loose from stretching and relaxed from a round of meditation before you begin.

Now that you're informed and prepared let's take a look at some advanced techniques!

I have noted every advanced pose with an indicative difficulty level system — 1 star being the easiest ones, to 5 stars for the most advanced ones - in case you want to escalate from the most basic ones to the most advanced.

Archer Pose (★★★★☆)

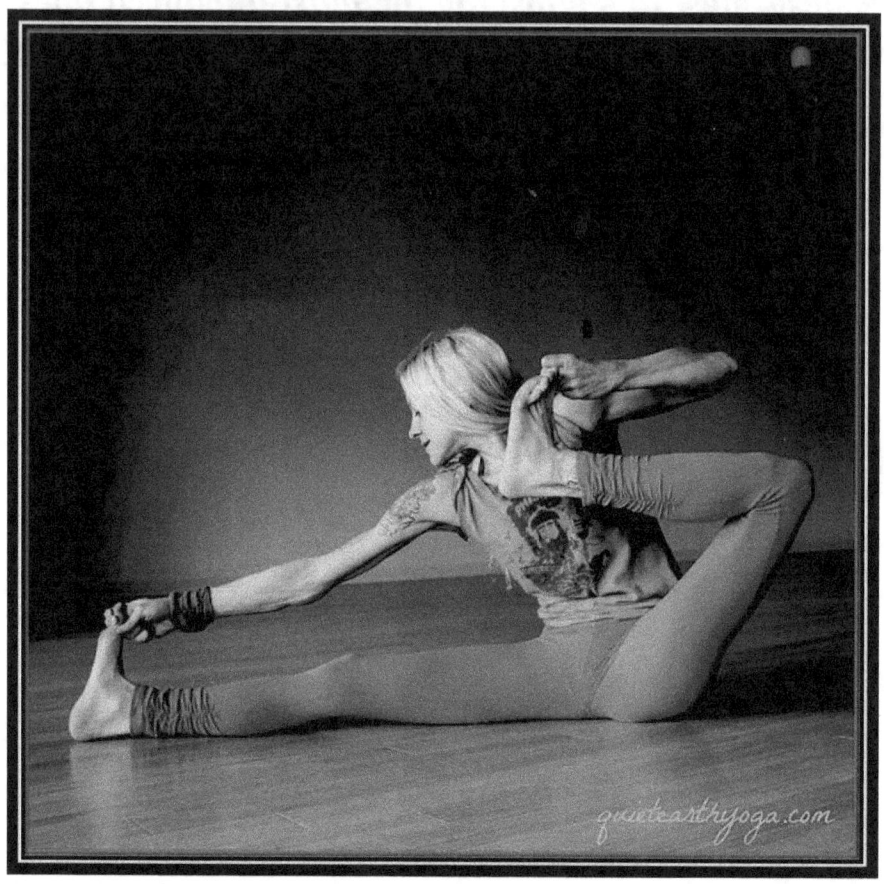

Photo courtesy of Amy at Flickr.com

The archer pose will strengthen your arms, abs, and back, and it will stretch those hamstrings as well as your calves.

1. To begin, sit in the staff position with your legs extended in front of you and your back straight. Reach forward and grab a hold of your toes and bend your knees gently if you have to in order to keep your back from rounding.

2. Exhale and use your right hand to pull your right foot close to your torso as you bend your knee. Keep your left arm and leg in their original positions. If you feel that this is enough, stay in this position.
3. If you feel you can go further, bring your right heel closer to your right ear and extend your lifted leg out as straight as you can.
4. To come out of the pose, exhale, and release your foot and extend it back to the floor.
5. Now do the other side!

★Preview End★

If you liked the preview you can download a copy of the book here